Natalia Montes Silva

Occupational Therapy in Critical Care Units

Natalia Montes Silva

Occupational Therapy in Critical Care Units

Role of the Occupational Therapist in the intervention of patients in Critical Care Units.

ScienciaScripts

Imprint

Cover image: www.ingimage.com

This book is a translation from the original published under ISBN 978-620-2-16386-6.

Publisher:
Sciencia Scripts
is a trademark of
Dodo Books Indian Ocean Ltd. and OmniScriptum S.R.L publishing group

120 High Road, East Finchley, London, N2 9ED, United Kingdom
Str. Armeneasca 28/1, office 1, Chisinau MD-2012, Republic of Moldova, Europe
Printed at: see last page
ISBN: 978-620-7-07956-8

OCCUPATIONAL THERAPY IN CRITICAL CARE UNITS

INDEX

INTRODUCTION

The health system in Chile is classified into different levels of complexity, these are the primary level, which is characterised by its low complexity but wide coverage, where mainly outpatient care is provided and where basic health programmes are carried out. The secondary level is of medium complexity and with a wide coverage, where the diagnoses and treatments of patients who could not solve their health problems in the primary level are carried out, and where both outpatient and inpatient care is provided. The last level is the tertiary level, which is highly complex and has low coverage, and is characterised by its high technological complexity and highly specialised human resources. It receives patients both from its own health care network and from other levels of care (Estructura y funcionamiento del sistema de salud chileno, 2019). To fulfil this function, it has a Critical Patient Unit (UPC), which is intended for the admission of seriously ill patients who need specialised clinical management to stay alive. It consists mainly of the intensive care unit (ICU) and the intermediate care unit (ICU) (Ministry of Health, 2017). In PCUs, there is a multidisciplinary approach where disciplines such as medicine, nursing and kinesiology have mainly formed these teams. However, in recent years, there has been an increase in the presence of occupational therapy (OT) in this area. This indicates how the contributions of this discipline have progressively positioned it in the health system. Another factor that is important to highlight is the importance that occupational therapy has gained since the current pandemic, recognising its importance in the treatment of patients hospitalised by COVID-19 as an indispensable part of the multidisciplinary team. One of the factors that has the greatest impact on the functionality of users who are admitted to the ICU is the time they spend bedridden and immobilised. For these patients, admission to the ICU means an indefinite period of hospitalisation due to the severity of their condition. In a study by Ruiz et al., 2016, it was found that the median length of stay in the ICU is 5 days, during which time functionality is diminished due to immobilisation and the use of mechanical ventilation, where its use fluctuates between almost 30% and 92% of patients admitted to the ICU (Ruiz et al., 2016).De Jonghe et al, 2002, identifies 3 variables that could have an impact on musculoskeletal alterations that affect functionality: number of days with dysfunction in at least 2 organs, use of corticosteroid treatment and gender. It is for this reason that early rehabilitation is of vital importance, as its objective is to prevent alterations in the musculoskeletal, neuromotor and cognitive systems (Celis, 2014). Studies support the feasibility and safety of rehabilitation in mechanically ventilated patients in intensive care (Celis, 2014), as it has a substantial impact on the maintenance of joint movement and strength, thus reducing the alteration of tissues that in the future could lead to permanent functional deterioration. In addition to the above, there are multiple studies that propose that mobilising the patient during periods without sedation reduces ventilation time, delirium and ICU stay (Celis, 2014). In this case, it is important to bear in mind that by reducing the probability or duration of delirium in patients, a factor that affects the suffering of transient or permanent neurological alterations is reduced (Tobar et al., 2019). It is possible to note that most of the existing protocols focus on re-establishing or maintaining structures in line with the Biomedical Reference Framework (Celis, et al 2014), where the functionality and performance of people in their occupations is not directly intervened. However, there are currently occupational therapists working in critical patient units, because the discipline is of great importance in the rehabilitation processes of patients in the PCU. Despite this, there are few protocols or clinical guidelines on the work of the occupational therapist in the hospital area of the critically ill patient. Taking into account the theoretical and practical basis of occupational therapy, it can be deduced that it could be an important contribution to the rehabilitation process of patients in the ICU. in the prevention of deterioration associated with critically ill patients, from prevention, early detection and early intervention, taking on a role that is not being developed by the unit's professional team (Celis, et. al 2014). One of the main functions of occupational therapy is to comprehensively assess and provide interventions according to the needs of each person through occupational diagnosis, selection, implementation and use of methods, techniques and resources relevant to each user, in order to improve their independence, especially in the maintenance of skills for the performance of their activities of daily living (Forsyth and Kielhofner, 2006).

HEALTH MODEL IN CHILE

The Chilean health model in 2003 presented a model of primary health care (PHC) defined in the International Conference on Primary Health Care (1978) as an integral part of the complete health care system, which contemplates promotion, prevention, treatment, rehabilitation and other sectors of national life; and privileging the highest participation of individuals and communities, encouraging responsibility in their health care, promoting teamwork and urging the most efficient use of available resources. After using this PHC model, the Ministry of Health (MINSAL, 2003) made a description of the Chilean Health Care Model, determining that as far as primary care is concerned, clinics do not have the capacity to solve the main health problems of the community. This is evidenced by deficiencies in the timeliness of care, affecting the population's impression of their reliability and generating problems in the way staff treat users. This would result in a high demand from the community for hospital emergency services (approximately 50% of total consultations) and excessive referrals from the clinic to the secondary level, with a lower level of resolution than expected for the primary level of care. It is stated that one of the areas for the transition of the care model should be "from the hospital axis to the secondary axis". The "primary health care system", as a result of epidemiological changes, is required to make an effort for the early detection and continuous care of people with chronic non-communicable diseases; primary health care being the place of care for the most prevalent pathologies, as well as being responsible for ensuring that people receive care of greater medical complexity when they really need it. To achieve these functions, it will have specialists and the appropriate technology to increase the required level of resolution, incorporated into a family health plan. It is for this reason that MINSAL (2004) postulates that PHC should develop the Comprehensive, Family and Community Health Model. This new health model is defined as the set of actions that promote and facilitate efficient, effective and timely care that addresses, rather than the patient or the disease as isolated facts, people, considered in their physical and mental integrity and as social beings belonging to different types of family and community, who are in a permanent process of integration and adaptation to their physical, social and cultural environment, i.e. a model of comprehensive health care with a family and network approach (Artaza et al., 2016).As stated by Becerril (2011) in his article on Chile's health system, the public sector is made up of all the bodies that make up the National Health Services System. (SNSS), which includes the Ministry of Health and its dependent agencies, the Institute of Public Health, the Central Supply Office, the National Health Fund (FONASA) and the Superintendence of Health. This sector covers approximately 70% of the population, including people in rural and urban areas, the lower middle class and pensioners, as well as professionals and technicians with higher incomes who choose to join it. The public sector is financed by general taxes, compulsory contributions and co-payments that are pooled in FONASA. Public services are provided by the SNSS, with its network of Regional Health Services, and the Municipal Primary Health Care System. The private sector is financed mainly by compulsory contributions collected in the Instituciones de Salud Previsional (ISAPRE), which cover approximately 17.5% of the population belonging to higher income social groups. In parallel, three mutuals offer protection to their members (15% of the population) against occupational accidents and diseases. The mutuals provide care in their own facilities. Chileans can choose between FONASA or an ISAPRE. The latter provide services in their own facilities, in other facilities in the same private sector or even in public sector facilities. Depending on the contracts, affiliates may or may not have a choice of service providers. A small section of the population, belonging to the upper class, makes direct out-of-pocket payments to private health care providers. About 10% of the population is covered by other public agencies, mainly the Armed Forces Health Services. The self-employed can choose to be affiliated to FONASA or an ISAPRE, or to be part of the population that is not affiliated to any social security health system.

On the other hand, in addition to these two sectors, the Ministry of Health (2020) establishes that the health care network is organised into primary care, which is the first level of contact with citizens, comprised of establishments that perform outpatient care functions in a given territory with a population under their care, such as health centres (CES), family health centres (CESFAM), community family health centres (CECOSF), rural health posts (PSR), Primary Emergency Care

Service (SAPU), High-Resolution Primary Emergency Care Service (SAR). And secondary care, which is provided by hospitals, institutes and diagnosis and treatment centres (CDT). If a person has been treated at the primary level and the health professional who has assessed him or her determines that he or she requires more complex care, the patient is referred to a specialised clinic or hospital.

Hospitals in the Chilean health system are mainly classified according to their contractual quality and their level of capacity. According to their contractual quality, there are two types of administrative dependence. Firstly, self-managed network hospitals, which are more technically complex and have a higher level of capacity and capacity to respond to the needs of their patients. as they include the development of specialties and an administrative organisation, they are decentralised but their care function is determined by the service director according to requirements. Secondly, hospitals of lower complexity, which depend on the health service to which they belong and their role is determined by the corresponding network.

According to what was recently presented by the Ministry of

Health (2020), there are three levels of resolution capacity:

- Low complexity hospitals: They bring health care closer to the population, mainly in extreme and highly rural areas. They cover the entire population in their jurisdiction with low complexity services and depend administratively on the Health Service to which they belong.

- Medium complexity hospitals: These are reference centres that provide coverage to the population within their jurisdiction. They depend administratively on the Health Service to which they belong.

- High complexity hospitals: They provide coverage to the entire population of the health service for high complexity services, mainly for critical patient units (UPC), according to the portfolio of services defined by the network manager. They can be self-managed and offer various specialties according to their function.

Structure of highly complex facilities

Within the organisational structure of highly complex facilities, the internal organisation of the facility is headed by the director of the facility, whose functions range from exercising the activities, regulation and standardisation of the management structure of the health care facility. The purpose of the director is to plan, direct, coordinate, coordinate, supervise and evaluate the management of the health care facility. In addition to the director in the internal organisation, there is also a sub-directorate for administrative management, care management, human resources management, operational management and finally the management of the outpatient and inpatient clinics.

This directory has internal advisory teams such as the User Management Unit, Planning and Management Control and the Communications and Public Relations Unit, Internal Audit, Legal Advice, Quality and Patient Safety, Hospital Infections, Epidemiological Surveillance, Information Security and Teaching and Care Relations (Servicio de Salud de Coquimbo, n.d.). The sub-directorate of Clinical Management of Closed Care has the function of contributing to providing comprehensive care to the user. It maintains constant coordination with the healthcare network to achieve effective continuity of care. Among its objectives is the efficient administration of care resources in terms of beds, supplies and human and technological resources. It also has closed surgical care services, such as hospitalisations (Servicio de Salud de Coquimbo, n.d.). Within this sub-directorate is the area of the Critical Patient Unit, both adult and paediatric.

Critical Patient Unit

The Critical Patient Unit (CPU), a structure that brings together the Intensive Care Unit and Intermediate Care Unit of a facility under a common organisation and unit for the care of critical patients (MINSAL, 2017). The PCU is a highly complex service whose objective is to ensure the survival of critically ill patients. These patients may arrive at the unit after a postoperative period, due to respiratory failure requiring ventilatory support, circulatory instability or shock, requiring constant monitoring and/or the use of special therapies such as vasoactive drugs (Tomicic, 2012).

Intensive Care Unit

The ICU corresponds to the hospital unit designed to provide medical, nursing, kinesiology and other necessary professional care to unstable critical patients, but with the possibility of recovery, in an effective, timely and permanent manner 24 hours a day, 365 days a year. This unit is is characterised by a concentration of highly trained staff, with permanent medical residency, as well as technology appropriate to its complexity (MINSAL, 2017). Furthermore, according to the American Association for Critical Care (AACI), critical care is medical care for patients whose illness requires close and constant monitoring by a team of specially trained caregivers. The AACI also defines the team of professionals involved in the rehabilitation process, which consists of:

Intensivist	A physician who has studied, trained and tested in the care of very ill patients. The intensivist is usually an expert in areas such as surgery, internal medicine, paediatrics and anaesthesiology.
Intensive care nurse	Highly trained nurse providing all aspects of care to a very sick patient.
Pharmacist	A drug expert who works with the care team toprescribe the medicines
	needed by the patient. The pharmacist checks the progress of these medicines during the patient's stay in hospital.
Dietician	The registered dietitian works with the care team and family to improve the health of the nutrient-deficient patient. The registered dietitian may direct or perform feeding by mouth, tube or vein.

Respiratory therapist	Professional trained in respiratory rehabilitation of hospitalised patients. The respiratory therapist uses pulmonary treatments to help the patient breathe.
Physiotherapist	Professional who helps to restore a body function involving muscles, bones, tissues or nerves. With this help, the patient is able to move better in daily life (e.g, walking, going up and down stairs).
	The physiotherapist uses techniques such as stretching and applying heat. These techniques can reduce pain and swelling. They can also prevent permanent physical disability.
Occupational therapist	A caregiver who helps the patient relearn life skills. Examples of these skills include hygiene, feeding, dressing, among others. The occupational therapist helps the patient to live as independently as possible.
Physician assistant or nurse practitioner	A caregiver trained and licensed in clinical services. He/she works in the ICU under the direction of the physician and performs actions such as taking the patient's medical history, ordering and interpreting medical tests and performing medical procedures.
Paediatrician	The child life specialist provides play therapy and distraction. He or she often works with other experts in the paediatric intensive care unit to improve the health and well-being of very ill children.

Intermediate Treatment Unit

The ICU corresponds to the hospital unit intended for the management of stable critically ill patients. It may exist exclusively in hospitals that do not require an ICU, in which case it must have a pre-established transfer network and a pre-transfer stabilisation or resuscitation bed. Where it coexists with an ICU, it will be an integral part of the CCU, constituting a single clinical and administrative unit (MINSAL, 2017).

Critically ill patient

The critical patient is defined by the American Society of Intensive Care Medicine as a patient who is physiologically unstable, requiring advanced life support and close clinical evaluation with continuous adjustments of therapy according to evolution.According to the most recent definitions of MINSAL (2017), the critical patient is a patient whose pathological condition affects one or more systems, which puts his or her life at serious actual or potential risk and who presents conditions of reversibility that require the urgent application of surveillance, monitoring, management and, eventually, advanced life support techniques. Furthermore, according to Tomicic (2012), for a patient to be considered a critical patient, he or she must meet the following inclusion criteria:

According to vital signs	Pulse <40 or > 150 beats per minute
	Systolic blood pressure< 80 mmHg or 20 mmHg below the patient's usual pressure
	Pressure blood mean < 60 mmHg.
	Diastolic blood pressure > 120 mmHg.
	Frequency respiratory rate >35 breaths per minute.
According to laboratory values	Serum sodium <110 mEq/L or > 170 mEq/L.
	Serum potassium <2 mEq/L or > 7 mEq/L.
	PaO2 < 50 torr (6.67 kPa).
	PH <7.1 or >7.7.
	Glycaemia > 800 mg/dL.
	Calcaemia > 15 mg/dL.
	Toxic drug or other chemical levels in a neurologically or haemodynamically compromised patient.
Inclusion criteria from imaging	Cerebrovascular haemorrhage.
	Contusion.
	Subarachnoid haemorrhage with altered consciousness or neurological focality.
	Ruptured viscera, bladder, liver, oesophageal varices, uterus, with circulatory instability.
	Dissecting aneurysm of the aorta.
Inclusion criteria according to electrocardiogram results	Myocardial infarction with complex arrhythmias.

	Instability haemodynamic instability or congestive heart failure.
	Arrhythmias supraventricular arrhythmias with haemodynamic instability.
	Sustained ventricular tachycardia or ventricular fibrillation.
	Complete AV block.
Inclusion criteria according to acute onset physical signs	Anisocoria plus altered consciousness.
	Burns greater than 10 % of the body surface.
	Anuria.
	Airway obstruction.
	Coma state.
	Status convulsus.
	Cyanosis.
	Cardiac tamponade.

REHABILITATION IN CRITICALLY ILL PATIENTS

Patients who are cared for in the critical patient unit, whether stable or unstable, require different types of management and eventually life support. Requirements range from pharmacological support and low-complexity devices to complex support through organ-supporting equipment (MINSAL, 2017).As mentioned, a multidisciplinary team works within the critical patient unit, composed of an intensivist, intensive care nurse, pharmacist, dietician, respiratory therapist, physiotherapist, occupational therapist, medical assistant or nurse practitioner and paediatrician, whose objective is to meet the needs of the patient's condition, as well as the requirements arising from their state of health, the level of complexity of their management and existing risk factors.The use of life support used in a large percentage of patients in the CPU involves immobilisation time that is required by this equipment. One of the most frequent complications in the PICU is ICU-acquired weakness, which is characterised by a decrease in muscle strength, generally associated with atrophy, of acute, diffuse, symmetrical and generalised onset, and whose aetiology is multifactorial and related to various risk factors, such as prolonged mechanical ventilation, stay in the ICU, prolonged immobility, use of neuromuscular blocking agents or corticotherapy, hyperglycaemia, shock, sepsis, renal failure (Celis, 2014). In addition to the above, a high percentage (+50%) of limb oedema has been identified. On the other hand, another of the most frequent alterations in the ICU is Delirium, a clinical condition of acute onset and fluctuating course, characterised by alterations in consciousness, attention and thinking. This occurs in a high percentage of patients admitted to the unit, reaching between 60% to 80% in patients under sedation with mechanical ventilation (Henao, 2013). Other factors associated with the condition include: sensory deficit, immobilisation, use of medications (sedatives, anticholinergics, polypharmacy, alcohol or drug withdrawal), acute neurological diseases, intercurrent diseases, metabolic disorder, surgery, clinical environment, pain, emotional distress and sleep deprivation (Celis, 2014). Taking this into consideration, patients not only need treatment for the pathology for which they are admitted to the PCU, but also the intervention of functional aspects that prevent sequelae at discharge through early rehabilitation.The rehabilitation of patients admitted to the UPC is based on interdisciplinary work. The aim is to provide early, minimally invasive and tolerable treatment, which focuses on intervention for the preservation of structures and functions that are intact, as well as those that have been affected both by the pathology and by the sequelae of the treatments provided in the unit.

OCCUPATIONAL THERAPY AT UPC

The occupational therapist in the health area promotes well-being, prevents impairments or disabilities and provides services to people with biological, psychological and social integration problems (Moreno et al., 2017). According to the Interdisciplinary Consensus on Rehabilitation for Adults Post COVID-19, at UPC level the intervention of Occupational Therapy is fundamental, as it has the theoretical and practical bases for helping to prevent much of the deterioration associated with the condition of the critical person, through timely detection and early intervention, actively participating in early mobilisation protocols, prevention of delirium, humanisation of care, among other functions. For the Hospital Clínico de la Universidad de Chile (Gallegos, n.d.) the objectives of occupational therapy in the critical patient unit are oriented to:

- To promote the maximum possible functionality necessary for the performance of activities of daily living.
- To increase the patient's ability to interact with the objects and people around him/her.

- To provide human and technical physical care necessary for the maintenance of body structures.

According to COPTOCAM, in terms of assessment, the occupational therapist as a member of the interdisciplinary team assesses the patient's progress throughout hospitalisation and continuation of rehabilitation with the aim of reducing the length of hospital stay as much as possible. In parallel, in the study "Occupational therapy in the intensive care unit" (Moreno et al., 2017), assessments associated with delirium in hospitalised persons, activities of daily living, mobilisation and pain, physical, cognitive and behavioural deficits, environmental and contextual assessment, and memory, perception and cognition are mentioned.With respect to the American Occupational Therapy Association (30) framework, it was found that the assessment process in the ICU is more related to the identification of the person's condition, in relation to the limiting factors in their health and participation (Moreno et al., 2017). In terms of intervention, COPTOCAM mentions that rehabilitation in the ICU takes place gradually, increasing in intensity day by day and taking into account the patient's circumstances, following the recommendations of the medical team where within the interventions incorporated it is recommended to incorporate a functional, cognitive and quality of life assessment as part of the patient's discharge report, as well as early mobilisation and the implementation of prevention and treatment measures.In the context of the UPCs, patients, according to their health situation, present an impact on occupations because there is an affectation in the client factors mainly in the structures, body functions and performance skills. such as motor and processing. Furthermore, hospitalisation and immobilisation processes exist in these, which, according to the aforementioned studies by Ohtake (2018) and Wilches (2018), have an impact on the occupational performance of critically ill patients, with one of the most affected occupations being ADLs related to self-care such as feeding, dressing, bathing, continence and transfer, with up to 35% dependence in some of these activities. The World Health Organisation (WHO), through the International Classification of Disability and Health Functioning (2001), defines dependence as "the situation in which a person with a disability requires assistance, technical or personal, for the performance (or improvement of functional performance) of a given activity". According to the aforementioned research, in UPCs, there is an impact on ADLs, thus generating dependency in these activities, since people require some kind of support to perform them. From an occupational therapy perspective, this need for support arises from the ineffective use of the performance skills required to perform these activities (AOTA, 2020).

SCIENTIFIC EVIDENCE

1. Occupational therapy and the critically ill patient (Celis, et al., 2014).

This study was conducted in the Adult Critical Care Unit of the Hospital Clínico de la Pontificia Universidad Católica de Chile (UPC-HCPUC), during 2012, where the characteristics of the critical patient were explored to obtain a global health profile during their stay in the UPC, in order to determine whether it would be possible to carry out an intervention from Occupational Therapy that would be a contribution to this unit. A prospective, observational study was carried out in the medical-surgical PCU for 25 days.

The results obtained allowed us to characterise the critical patient in this unit as a subject with a high probability of presenting compromised consciousness, oedema in the hand, limited range of joint movement (ROM) in the wrist and fingers, and a lack of stimuli that evoke their reality prior to hospitalisation.Finally, based on the analysis of the profile of the critical patient at the UPC-HCPUC and the context to which he/she is exposed, it is concluded that early Occupational

Therapy intervention could reduce and prevent the appearance of some signs associated with the critical patient, proving the hypothesis that, given the characteristics of this patient, it would be possible to carry out an Occupational Therapy intervention.

2. Functional independence in adult patients at discharge from intensive and intermediate care units (Wilches et al,. 2018).

Summary

The consequences of weakness acquired in the intensive care unit are manifested in functional dependence that makes it difficult to carry out activities of daily living. Objective: To describe changes in functional independence in adult patients discharged from the ICU and intermediate care (NICU). Methods: Descriptive study using retrospective information from physiotherapy records where data were collected on the level of functional independence assessed by the Barthel index at two points in time: at discharge from the ICU and at discharge from the NICU. Results: A total of 960 records were reviewed, of which 76 were included in the analysis. The mean age was 62 years, 38% were women and 62% were men. The average ICU stay was 3.4 days; 82.9% of patients admitted to the NICU were from the ICU of the same institution. Of 63 records of patients discharged from the ICU, 20.6% had total dependency and 47.6% severe dependency, while in NICU discharges only 3.2% had total dependency and 28.6% severe dependency. Regardless of the origin of the patients, upon discharge from NICU there was a 15-point increase in the IB, increasing from 30 to 45 points, a statistically significant change ($p<0.0001$). Conclusion: Significant changes in functionality were identified at ICU discharge compared to NICU discharge. Mechanical ventilation >48 hours had an impact negatively on the Barthel score, compromising activities of daily living such as grooming, dressing and ambulation.

3. Occupational therapy in intensive care units (Moreno et al., 2017).

Summary

Introduction. Since its inception, occupational therapy has been active in in-hospital settings. Currently, one of the goals for the consolidation of fields of knowledge, attention and prospective is to deepen the intervention carried out by the respective professional in the intensive care unit (ICU). Objective. To show the scientific evidence of occupational therapy intervention in an adult ICU through a literature review between 2010 and 2015, during which the categories of assessment, intervention modalities and outcomes were analysed. Materials and methods. Mixed research study, which seeks to specify the theoretical and practical sources that relate the terms of the research. In addition, a selective analysis process was carried out based on interests and significance. Results. Occupational therapy characterises activities based on mobilisation, positional changes, activities of daily living, stimulation, splinting, assistive technology, among others; it also brings benefits such as reduced length of stay, complications and costs. Conclusions. The importance of the work of the occupational therapist in the adult ICU is evident, as benefits such as reduced length of stay and functional improvement of people at the time of discharge are clear in international research.

4. Recommendations of the Chilean Society of Intensive Care Medicine for Analgesia, Sedation, Delirium and Neuromuscular Blockade in Adult Medical-Surgical Critically Ill Patients (Tobar et al., 2019).

Summary

Critically ill patients commonly develop pain and anxiety due to their clinical condition and/or the interventions and procedures necessary for their care, and for this reason the administration of analgesics and hypnotics is common in the CCU. The use of an appropriate strategy for the use of analgesia and sedation has been shown to improve clinical outcomes. The use of neuromuscular blockers has the potential to offer benefits to well-selected critically ill patients; however, they may be associated with ICU-acquired muscle weakness. Delirium has a high incidence in critically ill patients on mechanical ventilation, and is an independent predictor of adverse short- and long-term outcomes. Prevention strategies and early identification may offer an opportunity to improve patient outcomes. In consideration of the importance of this important topic, the

Chilean Society of Intensive Care Medicine (SOCHIMI) set out to develop an operational document with practical suggestions and recommendations applicable to our population. These suggestions and recommendations were made based on a structured analysis of the available evidence, other published guidelines on the subject and the experience of a multidisciplinary group of critical care professionals.

5. Role of Occupational Therapy in the Intensive Care Unit in Colombia (Moreno, Cubillos and Duarte, 2019).

Summary

In this study, the purpose of the research focuses on recognising and analysing occupational therapy intervention in intensive care units in Colombia. This is because it is necessary to have updated and detailed information on the processes and how they are carried out within the unit, in order to have a positive impact on the health, wellbeing and quality of life of the population admitted to an ICU. Through the collection of qualitative and quantitative data, the aspects analysed are oriented to learn about: participation, experience, evaluation, intervention and challenges of occupational therapy professionals. The results obtained from the research in the areas mentioned above show that the profession, within the area of early rehabilitation, is in an initial process of development, thus emphasising the need for further research. In terms of the interventions provided by a team that includes occupational therapists in its team, the results point to significant improvements. The challenge for the future is to deepen research and the publication of experiences and interventions that will lead to established protocols and guidelines to strengthen knowledge in the practice of rehabilitation in critically ill patients.

BIBLIOGRAPHY

Aguilera, X., Castillo, C., Covarrubias, T., Delgado, I., Fuentes, R., Gómez, M. I.,& Soto, M. (2019). Structure and functioning of the Chilean health system. Population Health Series No. 2.

Álvarez, E., Garrido, M., González, F., Guzmán, E., Donoso, T., Gallegos, S., Vergara, S., Aranda, R., Prieto, S., Briceño, C., Tobar, E., Alzamora, C., Bolvarán, C., Concha, C., Valencia, F., & Villalobos, F. (2012). Early and intensive occupational therapy in the prevention of delirium in older adults admitted to critical patient units. Randomized clinical trial: preliminary results. Revista Chilena de Terapia Ocupacional, 12(1), p. 44-59.

Álvarez, Garrido, Tobar, Prieto, Vergara, Briceño, González. (2016) Occupational therapy for delirium management in elderly patients without mechanical ventilation in an intensive care unit: A pilot randomized clinical trial, Journal of Critical Care Volume 37. p. 85- 90.

Arguelles, R. (2021). Hospital stay and rehabilitation of adult patients in the Intensive Care Unit of the Cayetano Heredia Hospital in the period 2018 to 2019. Peruvian University of Cayetano Heredia. Retrieved from:

https://repositorio.upch.edu.pe/handle/20.500.12866/9314

Artaza, O., Barría, M. S., Fuenzalida, A., Núñez, K., Quintana, A., Vargas, I., & Vidales, A. (2016). Modelo de gestión de establecimientos hospitalarios. Santiago: Ministry of Health.

American Occupational Therapy Association (2020). Framework for Occupational Therapy Practice: Domain and Process (Fourth Edition).edition). https://www.studocu.com/cl/document/universidad- santo-tomas-chile/areas-de-la-ocupacion/other/aota-2020-en-espanol-revisada-y-correcida/14508047/view

Becerril-Montekio, V., Reyes, J. D. D., & Manuel, A. (2011). Chile's health system. Salud pública de México, 53, s132-s142.

Celis, F., Gálvez, C., Moretti, C., Navarrete, E., Rovegno, M., & Torrent, V. (2014). Occupational therapy and the critically ill patient. Revista Chilena de Terapia Ocupacional, 14(1), pp. 101-110.

Interdisciplinary Consensus on Rehabilitation for Adults Post COVID-19 (2020). Recommendations for clinical practice.

De Jonghe, B., Sharshar, T., Lefaucheur, J., Authier, F., Durand-Zaleski, I., & Boussarsar, M. et al. (2002). Paresis

Acquired in the Intensive Care Unit A Prospective Multicenter Study. Journal Of The American Medical Association, (22).

Díaz (2011). The observation. Faculty of Psychology UNAM. Retrieved from http://www.psicologia.unam.mx/documentos/pdf/publicaciones/La_observacion_Lidia_Diaz_Sanjuan_Texto_Apoyo_Didactico_Metodo_Clinic_3_Sem.pdf

Forsyth, K. and Kielhofner, G. (2006). The human occupation model. Foundations for occupational therapy practice, 69-107.

Gallegos, S. (S.f) Strategies of occupational therapy intervention in critical patient unit: Evaluation and intervention of occupational therapy at UPC [Slide from PowerPoint]. Department of Occupational Occupational Therapy University of Chile. Retrieved from https://www.serviciodesaludaconcagua.cl/index.php/funcionarios/pack/ category/120-2019-ccurso-cambio-cambio-de-paradigma-de-los-cuidados-de- upc?download=731:2019-ccurso-cambio-de-paradigma-de-los-cuidados-de-upc.

Garzón, N., González, J. and Rojas, E. (2018). Proposal for improvement in ergonomic risk conditions associated with manual handling of patients in the Palliative Care Unit UCP presentes S.A.S. Bogotá, Colombia.

Guerrero Bejarano, M. (2016). Qualitative Research. INNOVA Research Journal, 1(2), 1-9. doi: 10.33890/innova.v1.n2.2016.7.

Hernández Aguado, S. (2014). Intervention of the occupational therapist in the area of cognitive stimulation. Psychiatric Inf., 137-145.

Hernández, R., Fernández, C. and Baptista, P. (2014). Metodología de la investigación. Mexico: Mc Graw Hill/ Interamericana Editores S.A.

Hoyos, S., García, R., Chavarro-Carvajal, D. and Heredia, R. (2015) Pressure ulcers in hospitalised patients. Bogotá, Colombia. Retrieved de: https://repositorio.comillas.edu/xmlui/handle/11531/36153.

Izcara Palacios, S (2014). MANUAL OF RESEARCH QUALITATIVE. Mexico City: Fontamara.

Jofré, A., Marshall, G., Rodríguez, A., Badal, M., Cabrera, G., Canals, M.,Paredes, F (2021).Critical pandemic situation: High levels of infection and hospitalisation in the country. ICOVID. Retrieved from: https://www.icovidchile.cl/.

Ministry of Health. (2020). Ministry of Health: Structure and

Functions. www.saludresponde.minsal.cl. Retrieved 20 July 2021,fromhttps://saludresponde.minsal.cl/wp-content/uploads/2020/11/Estructura-Minsal-EPT.pdf.

Ministry of Health, Redes Asistenciales, S. (2017). Norms for the organisation and operation of Paediatric Critical Patient Units (UPCP).

Ministry of Health. Transition to the Networked Care Model. Santiago, Chile, 2003.

Ministry of Health (2004). División de Gestión de la Red Asistencial, Departamento de Atención Primaria. Modelo de atención integral - familiar-comunitario y redes asistenciales. Unidad Modelo de Atención. Santiago, Chile.

Miralles, P. (2017). Conceptual principles of occupational therapy. Madrid: Síntesis.

Monje Álvarez, C. (2011). RESEARCH METHODOLOGY QUANTITATIVE AND QUALITATIVE: Teaching guide. Surcolombiana University.

Moreno-Chaparro, J., Cubillos-Mesa, C., & Duarte-Torres, S. C. (2017). Occupational therapy in intensive care unit. Revista de la Facultad de Medicina, 65(2), 291-296.

Moreno-Chaparro, J., Cubillos-Mesa, C., & Duarte-Torres, S. C. (2019). Role of Occupational Therapy in the Intensive Care Unit. in Colombia. Revista Ciencias de la Salud, 17(1), 70. https://doi.org/10.12804/revistas.urosario.edu.co/revsalud/a.7614

Morrison, D. (2011) (Re)meeting the founders and "mothers" of occupational therapy. An approach from feminist studies on science. TOG (A Coruña). Retrieved from: http://www.revistatog.com/num14/pdfs/original4.pdf.

Ohtake, PJ, Lee, AC, Scott, JC, Hinman, RS, Ali, NA, Hinkson, CR, ... and Smith, JM (2018). Physical impairments associated with post-intensive care syndrome: systematic review based on the world health organization international classification of functioning, disability and health framework. Physiotherapy , 98 (8), 631- 645. Retrieved from: https://doi.org/10.1093/ptj/pzy059.

Okuda, M. and Gómez-Restrepo, C. (2005). Methods in qualitative research: triangulation. Revista Colombiana de Psiquiatría, 34(1), 118-124.

World Health Organization. (2001). International classification of functioning, disability and health. Retrieved from: https://aspace.org/assets/uploads/publicaciones/e74e4-

cif_2001.pdf.

Pereira, A., Ruiz, M. and Suarez, D. (2009). Proposal of equipment, materials and basic instruments for the operation of occupational therapy services in hospital settings in the area of physical dysfunctions. Bogotá, Colombia. National University of Colombia.

Quiroz O, T., Araya O, E., & Fuentes G, P. (2014). Delirium: update in non-pharmacological management. Revista chilena de neuro- psiquiatría, 52(4), 288-297. https://d o i . org/10.4067/s0717-92272014000400007.

Tog. magazine (2014). Evolution of the philosophy of occupational therapy from its beginnings as a profession. Retrieved from: http://revistatog.com/num20/pdfs/historia1.pdf.

Riemann, B., Lephart, S. (2003). The Sensorimotor System, Part I: The Physiologic Basis of Functional Joint Stability. Journal of Athletic Training. 37(1), 71-79.

Rubio Ortega C, Berrueta Maetzu LM, Duran Castillo P. (2004). Evaluation of occupational therapy from its beginnings as a profession. TOG.

Ruiz, C., Díaz, M. Á., Zapata, J. M., Bravo, S., Panay, S., Escobar, C.& Castro, R. (2016). Characteristics and evolution of patients admitted to an Intensive Care Unit of a public hospital. Revista médica de Chile, 144(10), 1297-1304.

Schweickert, WD, Pohlman, MC, Pohlman, AS, Nigos, C., Pawlik, AJ, Esbrook, CL, ... and Kress, JP (2009). Early physical and occupational therapy in critically ill patients on mechanical ventilation: a randomised controlled trial. The Lancet , 373 (9678), 1874-1882.

Segovia Díaz de León, Martha Graciela, & Torres Hernández, Erika Adriana (2011). Functionality of the elderly and nursing care. Gerokomos, 22(4), 162-166. https://dx.doi.org/10.4321/S1134-928X2011000400003.

Society of critical care medicine. Available at: http://www.myicucare.org/Pages/default.aspx.Recuperado on 23 July, 2021.

Tobar, E., Rojas, V., Álvarez, E., Romero, C., Sepúlveda, I., & Cariqueo, M. et al. (2019). Recommendations of the Chilean Society of Intensive Care Medicine for Analgesia, Sedation, Delirium and Neuromuscular Blockade in Adult Medical-Surgical Critically Ill Patients. Revista Chilena De Medicina Intensiva, (3). Retrieved from https://medicina-intensiva.cl/revista/pdf/68/5.pdf.

Tomicic, V. (2012). Admission and Discharge to Intensive Care Units. Retrieved September 11, 2012, from Universidad Católica de Chile, Programa de Medicina Intensiva, website:http://escuela.med.puc.cl

Valencia (n/d). Documentary review in the research process. Retrieved from https://univirtual.utp.edu.co/pandora/recursos/1000/1771/1771.pdf.Willard, H., Spackman, C., Crepeau, E., Cohn, E. & Schell, B. (2005). Occupational therapy. Madrid Buenos Aires: Médica Panamericana.

Wilches-Luna, E., Méndez, A. and Gastaldi, AC (2018). Functional independence in adult patients at discharge from intensive and intermediate care units. Revista Chilena de Medicina intensiva , 33 (1), 7-14.

World Federation of Occupational Therapists (2012). About occupational therapy. Retrieved from https://www.wfot.org/about- occupational-therapy.

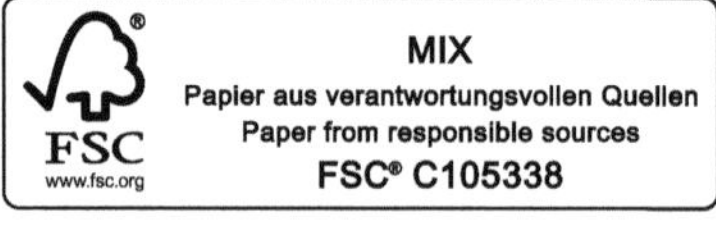

Printed by Books on Demand GmbH, Norderstedt / Germany